How to Make Your Baby Sleep

Contents

Introduction

I want to thank you and congratulate you for downloading the book. "How to Make Your Baby Sleep."

Raising a baby is no child's play. Right from taking care of the baby's food needs, to ensuring you all get a good night's sleep, new parents have their work cut out for them even before the baby arrives in the world.

It is vital for new parents to be proactive and prepare themselves for the journey into parenthood. They must plan everything out in such a way that allows them to enjoy every minute of the journey and experience immense joy. Whether you are just days away from giving birth, or have already welcomed your newborn into your lives, this book will serve as your sleep training guide.

The book has been designed to teach you how you can take care of your baby's needs and ensure that baby gets enough sleep during the growing years. Sleep remains an important aspect of baby's growth and development and this book will guide you through the process.

Thanks again for downloading this book. I hope that you enjoy it and that the information is useful to you.

Chapter 1 – The Importance of Sleep and Getting Started

Sleep is an extremely important part of life. It is that much more important for babies to get sleep as their bodies will be in the growth stages.

In this chapter, we look at the importance of sleep for babies.

Hormones

Hormones are one of the most important aspects of bodily growth. Hormones serve multiple functions in the body including promoting growth, enhancing cell function, encouraging good blood circulation and many other such important functions. One of the best ways to promote hormone health is through sleep. Your baby will require lots of sleep to keep his or her hormones in check. These will especially remain active at night and help your baby to grow in size.

Healing

Sleep induces healing properties. It is extremely important for your baby's body to repair itself from the inside out in order to achieve proper growth. Sleep can fix a whole host of issues including organ repair, tissue repair, dealing with colds and fevers, etc. It is, therefore, important for your baby to get enough sleep.

Ideal Weight

According to research studies done on infants, those babies who get less sleep per night are more likely to gain unhealthy weight. Sleep helps with the secretion of leptin, which is a hormone that signals fullness. If this hormone does not function properly, then your baby will start eating more and thus gain weight. It will therefore be important for your baby to get enough sleep during the night to prevent excess weight gain and obesity.

Mood Enhancement

Nobody likes a grumpy baby! As per studies, babies who do not sleep enough remain grumpy during their waking hours. There therefore means your baby should get enough sleep during the day, and also at night, in order to remain happy and healthy. If you have seen a baby who is grouchy, you will know that this isn't the best case scenario for either the parent or the baby.

Healthier Brain

Brain health is of vital importance. As per research studies, those babies who sleep more develop a healthier brain. A study was conducted with infants, where one set of babies was made to take a nap after being exposed to pictures and sounds while the other set of babies was encouraged to stay awake. It was found that the first group remembered things better than the second group. This goes to show that taking a nap helped the babies to consolidate the information after every successive sleeping session.

Getting Started with It

The very first step of the process will be to prepare yourself for the new situation. Many parents tend to forget about themselves and focus more on the baby's needs. While this is a natural reaction, you must make it a point to sleep as much as you can during the day, you need to prepare yourself mentally and physically so that you are able to take care of baby and yourself. This daytime nap will help you to settle in with your baby's sleeping schedule, as most babies tend to wake up during the night. You have to tell yourself that you will enjoy the journey and help your baby to have a great time growing up as well.

Pact

Both you and your partner will have to work on a pact to share the responsibilities of coping with the needs of your newborn. It is not just the mother's job to raise the baby and the father should be encouraged to put in equal effort. It will also be easier for the baby to fall asleep if he or she is accustomed to both parents. Make a list of responsibilities and divide them among yourselves. By doing this, you will have the chance to reduce the load and enjoy the experience between you.

Timetable

A timetable is a must when it comes to raising a baby. Not having one can make you feel overwhelmed and lead to panic. You have to make a table that lists clearly the times when you have to feed your baby, prepare his or her meals, prepare your meals, have your meals, put your baby to bed, schedule your own sleep, etc. Prepare a format and then fill in the details every day or every week. With time, you will get accustomed to it and settle in with a routine.

Lifestyle

New parents will have to undergo a few lifestyle modifications when they welcome their newborn into their home environment. You might not have the chance to go out as much or meet friends. You may also have to forego watching your favorite TV shows and indulging in other such regular activities or try recording programs to watch at other times. Remember that it will only be temporary and you do not have to abandon the activities that you love forever. You will be able to return to these activities once your baby grows a little older.

Seek Help

You can employ people to help you out with your routine activities in order to lessen your load. This could be a nanny or a cook or both. They can help you by taking away some of the extra work, ensuring you spend as much time as possible with your baby. You can also ask your parents or siblings to help out sometimes. Invite them over while you are still pregnant, as family is important at a time like this and they may volunteer without much persuasion.

Set up the Room

Some parents wait until the arrival of their baby to decide on a room and decorate it, thinking that they have plenty of time. However, it would be best to prepare in advance and have your baby's room decorated well in advance. Right from the décor to the lighting to the temperature, you have to ensure that everything is in good shape before baby's arrival. Apart from baby's room, you must also focus on setting up the entire house. Ensure that you are prepared for baby's arrival well in advance so you don't have extra worries at a time which is going to be stressful for you. You may need to consider how to keep pets away from the baby while baby sleeps.

Research

You must conduct as much research on the topic as possible in order to prepare yourself for the journey that lies ahead of you. Make it a point to read up on parenthood. This book will make a great guide, no doubt, but do not limit yourself to just this. Buy books on raising babies and learn how you can help your baby in other ways. Turn to the Internet and find sites that provide you with extensive information on the topic. Forums where parents get together may be a good idea as this gives you experienced parents who may be able to answer any questions you may have.

Buy Everything

Try to buy all your baby's supplies in advance. You will need diapers, lotions, bottles, bibs, etc. Buy them online in bulk and store them in baby's room so that they are easily available. Remember, baby will grow quickly so don't invest too much on first size clothing, however cute it may be.

Supplies

It will be important to buy all supplies in advance and keep them stocked up. As you know, baby may surprise you and arrive early. Some of these supplies include diapers, creams and lotions, etc. as mentioned above. Having these handy will ensure that you are able to tend to your baby on time and not affect his or her sleep cycle. Make a full list of the different things required and tick them off one by one. Ensure that you order everything and keep them neatly stacked in baby's room so that these items are easily available. Apart from the day to day supplies, you will also need to choose a crib, changing bag and other items.

Chapter 2 – Sleep Basics and Setting up the Room

Sleep is one of your baby's most important activities. It is normal for your newborn to sleep for between 10/14 hours a day. You have to encourage your baby to sleep as much as he/she can so that the baby gets all the benefits mentioned in an earlier chapter. It will be extremely important to establish good sleeping habits right from a young age. Your baby has to sleep during the day and at night, in order to develop a strong and healthy mind and body.

Sleep Basics

Bed

The first thing to set up for your baby is where the baby will sleep. In the early stages, this needs to be a safe environment. Small babies won't need a cot as this is used at a later stage, when the baby is larger.

- The crib should be soft to the touch and comfortable for your baby to sleep in. Choose cotton based bedclothes and make sure that there are no hard surfaces which may harm baby. The reason why cotton is used is because it does not cause the baby to itch.
- Get rid of any toys from the crib or other hanging objects that can loosen and fall inside the crib. Check that mobiles are at a safe distance from tiny hands.
- The crib should be placed low enough to prevent your baby from falling out of it.

- Check the cot (for toddlers) or crib to ensure that there is nothing that is sharp or potentially dangerous in the immediate area.
- If you plan on making your baby sleep in bed with you, then ensure that there is enough space for your baby to move around. It is not a good idea when you know that you are going to sleep as you may crush the baby.
- Do not place your baby in his or her sibling's bed.
- Bumper pads are unsafe for babies. You have to remove them if they are part of the crib.
- If the crib has castors, then ensure that the wheels are locked when the baby is inside the crib. If they are not, then this can pose a risk. Similarly, if you have a rocking crib, make sure that the rocking mechanism is locked in place especially as baby starts to get older.

Atmosphere

- The atmosphere inside the room should be comfortable for your baby. It should not be too hot or too cold. It is ideal to maintain the temperature at between 60 and 70 degrees Fahrenheit. If you are worried about it being too hot or cold, then be sure to look in on baby often. The cot or crib should be in the middle of the room during summer and certainly placed away from open doors and windows where there may be a draft. It should also be away from radiator as they can heat up easily and baby may burn his/her hands.
- During winters, keep the windows open during the mornings and close them at night. This will help with air circulation and allow your baby to sleep better. If there are any bad odors left from changing diapers, air the

room during the day, so the room can be warmed up ready for the baby's night time sleep.

- Do not use any room fresheners or sprays as that can irritate your baby's nasal passages. The room should be as quiet as possible and not exposed to loud noises from outside. Be aware of closing windows if there is a lot of noise outside.
- Babies get used to familiar sounds that are soothing. You can play a little light music to soothe your baby to sleep. You may even find a wind up musical bedside lamp will help but this must always be out of reach of the crib.
- When it comes to the lighting, try to block out at least 80 percent or the light so that your baby is not disturbed by it. A dim light can be left in the room so that you don't need to turn on a harsh light when baby needs you, but no light should be in baby's face or eyes. Switch off all overhead lights when your baby is sleeping.
- Use curtains and blinds to block off the light during the day.

Safety precautions

- Pick out all baby proof items for the baby's room. This includes toys, pillows, bed sheets, blankets and also blinds and curtains. Make sure that the paints you use in the room are baby friendly.
- Take away from baby's reach all creams, lotions, cosmetics, toiletries, etc. Babies can ingest them if left unattended.
- The cot or crib should be placed in a safe location. You have to push it as far away from the windows as possible, especially open windows.

- You will spend a lot of time with baby in the early days. It's always a good idea to have a comfortable chair in the nursery.

Chapter 3: Good Sleeping Habits from the Beginning

It will be extremely important to establish good sleeping habits right from the very beginning. As you are aware, what babies learn during the early stages of life is what will stick and it will be harder to correct bad habits later.

You must ensure that your baby develops positive habits from the moment baby comes home. Here are some tips that can help you establish good sleeping habits from a young age.

Identify what works best

It is no secret that every child is different. The first step in the process will be to identify what works best for your baby. This can include knowing what type of pacifier works best for him or her, what type of atmosphere the baby prefers to sleep in, whether your baby likes to be fed just before taking a nap or after waking, etc. You will have to undergo some level of trial and error to know exactly what suits your baby and stick with whatever works best. Maintain a journal and write down what works so that you can use it for future reference. You may need to give this information to a babysitter.

Routine

Nothing works better than following a set schedule or routine. When you follow a routine, you are instilling a routine into baby's life too. This will go a long way toward establishing good habits in your baby. You should make a timetable to feed your baby, put him or her to bed, establish a playtime, etc. Your baby's body will adjust to the timetable and make it easier for you to train the baby. Remember the different phases of growth and teething, etc. and this will need to evolve as the baby grows older.

Position

The sleep position you choose for your baby holds much significance. You have to ensure that baby is comfortable when asleep and not twisting and turning. For the first 12 months, you have to place your baby on his or her back. This is the safest position and minimizes the risk of SIDS. Once your baby is able to fall asleep on his or her own, then they can choose whatever position feels comfortable for them. You may wish to swaddle your baby in the early stages to ensure that the baby is safe.

Hygiene

It is vital to establish sleep time hygiene. You must ensure that the surroundings are clean and your own hands are clean before touching your baby. You will have to teach your toddlers the importance of washing and cleaning their teeth before going to bed. Bad hygiene can cause sleeping issues such as apnea. You must ensure that the crib is clean when putting baby to bed.

Naps

Naps are an extremely important part of your baby's sleeping routine. Babies have to sleep in the morning as this is important to their growth. You must encourage babies to nap in the mornings. Some babies can suffer from sleeplessness and require help from parents to fall asleep. You can rock baby to sleep or swaddle baby if this helps. It is natural for babies to sleep for 10 to 12 hours during the day, as their bodies will require ample rest. If your baby's circadian rhythm is off, then you should try to normalize it by getting them to sleep more at night and play with them in the mornings.

Stop Prompting

Your child should learn to fall asleep by him or herself. This should ideally happen at around toddler age. You can use the Ferber method which is a method to help baby sleep or get baby to fall asleep naturally. This is outlined later in the book.

Patience

You have to exercise some level of patience when it comes to teaching your baby to fall asleep. You must stay with the baby and ensure that the baby feels supported. Don't rush baby. Babies have to take their time to adjust to a new schedule.

Chapter 4 – Understanding the Baby's Psychology

Many people find it tough to understand babies and their behavior. This is especially true for new parents who are unable to make sense of why their baby is following a strange sleeping pattern. To help you with this process, we will look at some baby psychology basics:

Sleep patterns

Most babies will follow a strange sleeping pattern. Their circadian rhythm will not be adept to the concepts of night and day and babies frequently end up sleeping more during the day and less during the night. It can take anywhere from a couple of months to a year for them to get adjusted to the concepts of night and day.

Bays are light sleepers. They will not go into a state of deep sleep like most adults do. They will also not spend much time in REM phase or rapid eye movement phase. As parents, it will be best to identify a few sings that tell you whether your baby is sleepy.

- Check to see if your baby is yawning. That is the first sign that he or she is sleepy and wants to fall asleep,
- Check to see if your baby is rubbing his or her eyes. This is another sign that will tell you whether your baby is sleepy.
- Some babies scratch their ears as a sign that they are sleepy. They will mostly scratch the top end of their ears.
- Some babies develop dark circles under their eyes that

deepen when they are sleepy.

- If your baby is cranky, then he or she is sleepy.
- Some babies will stop responding to playfulness and simply stare without much reaction. This is indicative of the need to sleep.

As mentioned earlier, you have to train your baby right from a young age to develop positive sleeping habits. Here are some positive habits to instill when they are still babies. Following two different schedules for daytime and night time will work well with your baby. You will be able to help him or her to sleep correctly.

- One good way of teaching the difference between nighttime and daytime is by maintaining two different sets of clothing – one for day and one for night. Maintain colorful clothes for mornings and sleep clothes for nighttime. Change the baby as soon as baby wakes up and just before going to bed.
- Keep your baby as active as possible during the day. Talk to him or her and also play with the baby. Make the baby spend time in the living room or family room where there is activity.
- Mornings are a great time for friends and family members to visit and play with the baby.
- Open up all the windows and push aside the screens to allow light to seep into the room where the baby is during the day. The sound of traffic, people talking, etc., will all tell your baby that it is time for him or her to be awake.
- Talk to your baby as you feed him/her during the daytime. Tell baby stories and get baby to pay attention.
-

Night Time

- Try not to speak with your baby while feeding him/her at night. You must be as silent as possible.

- Close all the doors and windows and ensure that the room is dark and free of sounds.
- Yawn a few times so that your baby knows that it's time to sleep.
- Follow a nighttime routine that will signal to him or her that it is time to sleep.

These form the simple tricks to help your baby differentiate between daytime and night time.

Chapter 5 – Sleep Training from Newborn – 6 months old

Newborn babies require a lot of care and attention especially in regard to their meals and sleep. In this chapter, we will look at feeding and sleeping times to follow with your newborn baby.

Feeding your baby

- Your newborn baby will feed on milk quite frequently. Babies aged 3 to 6 months will have extremely small stomachs and so will have to be fed small amounts at regular intervals.
- Meals can refer to breast milk or formula food. Although breast milk should be the number one preference to feed babies with, some mothers choose formula if they are taking medications that can seep through breast milk.
- Babies easily digest breast milk, so you will have to feed more often. Formula, however, is not easily digested and therefore will have to be fed less frequently.
- Most babies will consume anywhere between 25 and 30 ounces of breast milk every day. Your baby should be fed every couple of hours so that the supply is consistent.
- A simply rule to follow to know how much formula to feed your baby is by multiplying your baby's weight by 2.5. Say, for example, your baby weighs 12 pounds. You will have to feed him or her 30 ounces of formula every day.
- Some babies can sleep for longer hours at a stretch. They might not wake up every couple of hours. In such cases, the mother may have to pump the milk using a pump and store it. That way, there will be a consistent supply of

breast milk for the baby.

- Some babies tend to sleep for 4 to 5 hours at a stretch. For such times, you can use a breast pump to pump out the milk and store it to feed the baby once your baby wakes up. If you are ready to feed baby, then simply discard the pumped milk that has not been used.
- Babies aged newborn to 6 months will eliminate food quite often. You must check every couple of hours and change their diapers as often as possible to prevent rashes and other issues.

Sleep Pattern

Newborn babies sleep quite a lot. This is normal as their bodies will still be growing and require sleep to ensure correct growth. Newborns will sleep for 19 to 20 hours per day. This will be spread across mornings, afternoons, evenings and nighttime.

If your baby was born at midnight or post-midnight, then chances are high that his or her circadian rhythm will be off. The circadian rhythm refers to your baby's sleep cycle. If it is out of whack, then your baby will stay awake during the nighttime and sleep during the day. You have to try and fix this as soon as possible, or else you will have to stay up at night frequently.

Let's take a look at your baby's sleep cycle.

No rapid eye movement

The no rapid eye movement or NREM phase is considered the most important phase of sleep. It is during this phase that growth hormones are released into the body. These hormones are responsible for your baby's growth and development. The blood supply to the body is highest during this phase and the muscles remain relaxed.

Rapid eye movement

The next phase is known as rapid eye movement or REM. During this phase, the mind remains a little alert and does not go into a state of deep sleep. Your newborn baby will sleep in this phase for the first month after birth.

Babies aged 3 to 6 months will sleep for shorter spells and wake up every 30 to 60 minutes. They will not be able to sleep for long hours as they will only sleep in the REN phase.

Babies at this age will automatically fall asleep every few minutes. You can pick a routine to help them fall asleep faster such as swaddling or rocking. Do stop rocking as soon as he or she falls asleep as otherwise, the baby's rhythm may be upset.

Chapter 6 – Sleeping Guide for 7-10 Month old Babies

Babies aged 7 to 10 months old will develop a different feeding and sleeping pattern altogether. They will also change their behavior and start adjusting to regular daytime and nighttime routines.

Feeding the Baby

Babies aged 7 to 10 months will gradually reduce the amount of milk they consume per day. This will be a good time to shift them to solid food.

The transition from milk to solid food can be quite difficult, as your baby's body will have to adjust to it. It will therefore be best to take it slowly so that your baby is able to adjust to the new diet.

A good way to introduce solid foods is by following the 4-day trial method. Using this method, you feed your baby some solid food and wait for at least 4 days to see how he or she reacts to it. If the baby is able to adjust to it then you can continue feeding them solid foods.

If you notice any allergic reaction then it is best to discontinue feeding the baby unfamiliar foods.

Fruits are best to start with. Feed your baby mashed bananas and wait for 4 days before feeding the baby another fruit. Start on a Monday morning and wait until Friday to introduce another fruit.

Continue this until your baby is around 10 months old, after which time, you can rest the 4 day rule.

You can check for some basic signs to know whether your baby is ready for solid foods. Here they are in detail:

- First off, check whether your baby is able to sit by him/herself on the high chair and eat food without your help. This will be indicative of your baby being ready for solid food.
- Next, check if your baby is readily accepting the food being offered to him or her. A baby should open its mouth to accept the food.
- Once baby is ready, give the baby just a small amount of solid food to check whether the baby is comfortable eating what you have given. If the baby hesitates, then make the quantity less.
- Be patient with your baby and ensure that you take it slowly. Doing too much at once can lead to problems and diarrhea.

Once babies have finished eating, they should be given fluids. Do not be in a hurry to put the baby down to sleep after eating. Leave a gap of at least 30 minutes.

At this stage, your baby will not eliminate as much as when he or she was younger. You can reduce the frequency of diaper changes.

Sleeping

Babies aged 7 to 10 months will sleep better and follow a predictable pattern. Their naps will not be as erratic as before, thereby helping parents to get some much-needed sleep.

- This stage is characterized by predictable sleeping routines. You will find that your baby is taking predictable naps during the day and sleeping a certain number of hours at night. This will help you fix your own sleeping schedule.
- At this stage, your baby will not want to be rocked or swaddled. The baby will try to fall asleep by itself and not like being prompted.
- In order to build on this habit, you must slowly reduce the rocking and patting and let your baby get used to falling asleep on his/her own.
- Your baby will typically sleep for around 15 hours a day. It will be much less than in the earlier days.
- Babies' bodies will be undergoing several changes at this stage in their life. Right from developing motor skills to enhancing cognition, they will experience a lot of mental and physical changes. This can make them a little restless and cranky at times. Parents are advised to gently handle babies at this age and rock them to sleep if this is found to help.
- Some babies will find it difficult to sleep on their own and want to sleep with their parents. If you have been co-sleeping and want your baby to have a different sleeping space, then now is not a good time to transition as babies of this age will already be undergoing stress.
- Babies aged 7 to 10 months old will enjoy developing a bedtime routine. They will be open to learning new things and getting them to develop a regular habit will help them to sleep better. This can include giving him or her a

bath, listening to rhymes together, etc. Your baby will
begin to associate the habit with the act of falling asleep.
- Parents need to avoid feeding babies before bedtime as
this may interfere with their ability to get off to sleep at
this age.
- Now will be a good time to set an appropriate sleeping
time for your baby. Your child will get used to this routine
and continue with it on an ongoing basis. It will be ideal
to put children of this age to bed by 8 as that way, they
can fall asleep by 8.30 pm.

Following this guide will help your baby develop good sleeping
habits that can last a lifetime.

Chapter 7 – Sleeping Guide for Babies aged 8-12 Months Old

Babies aged between 8 to 12 months will be ready to develop permanent sleeping habits. You can now successfully introduce them to a morning and nighttime routine that they can follow. Here is a simple feeding and sleeping guide that is suited to babies of this age range:

Timetable

By now, your baby will be completely used to eating solid foods. You will not have to put in as much effort to get them to develop the habit. Here is a daily timetable to follow with your baby:

- 7 am to 8 am: Your baby will be up by this time and you can feed him or her 7 to 8 ounces of milk or formula.
- 8 am to 9 am: Change your baby's clothes so that the baby is in day wear clothing.
- 8.30 am to 9 am: Give your baby finger foods to munch on. Your child can have whatever breakfast you consume on a routine basis including vegetable sticks, fruits, cereals, etc.
- 9 am to 10 am: Baby can play with toys or watch cartoons or read a book while you carry out your morning routine. Be sure not to let your baby out of your sight.
- 10 am: Feed your baby 7 ounces of breast milk or formula.
- 12 pm: Set a lunch for your baby consisting of light snacks that h or she can munch on. You can give your baby vegetables, fruits, meats or other such filling foods. Do not give your child junk food or processed foods.

- 12.30 to 3 pm: Your baby can play or read or listen to music. Ensure you stay with your baby and play with your child as much as possible.
- 3 pm to 6 pm: Take your baby out for a walk or to play with others. You can also take your baby out while you go shopping. Get your baby to take a nap at about the 4.30 mark and wake your baby up at 6 pm.
- 6 pm to 7 pm: Prepare a bath for baby by adding great smelling essential oils suitable for a baby. It will rejuvenate the baby's senses and make the baby happy and energetic.
- 7 pm to 8 pm: Give baby dinner. You can follow the same menu as the child had earlier or prepare something else. Follow it up with 7 to 8 ounces of breast milk or formula.
- 8 pm.: Put your baby in bed. Try not to rock or pat your baby to sleep. Babies find it easy to fall asleep if you read them a story and stay close by the bed with them.

You need not stick with the same routine and may come up with a guide of your own to follow that works for you and your child.

Sleeping routine

Babies aged 8 to 12 months will be able to sleep on their own without much effort. Bit it would still be best to follow a schedule as follows:

- As mentioned earlier, this will be a great time for you to follow routines, as they will stick with the baby for the foreseeable future. You can set an appropriate bedtime so that your baby can fall asleep at the same time every day.
- You will finally be able to have a full night's sleep, as your baby will sleep throughout the night. Your baby will stop feeding at night as well. Most babies at this age will sleep for 10 to 11 hours without a break in between naps. You

can adjust your sleeping hours accordingly.

- Your baby will not sleep so much during the daytime. He or she will take only a couple of predictable naps.
- Your baby will be quite active now, especially during mornings and evenings. Try to play with your baby as much as possible and read stories to your child.
- Reduce patting and rocking the baby and gradually stop this behavior. Your baby should get used to sleeping on its own without any help from you.
- Now will be a great time to move your baby to his or her own room or cot. Babies of this age find it easier to transition and prefer to sleep on their own.
- You can prepare a nice room for your baby and ensure the atmosphere is tailored to the child's needs. Right from the lighting to the temperature, ensure that everything is perfect for your baby. Stay with your baby until the baby gets accustomed to being in this room and falls asleep.

These form the simple steps to follow in order to sleep train your 8 to 12 month old baby.

Chapter 8 – Sleeping Guide for Babies Aged 13-18 Months

Babies aged between 13 and 18 months will be able to develop permanent eating and sleeping habits. They will also become quite independent. Here is a simple feeding and sleeping guide to follow:

Feeding guide

Now is a good time to sit with your baby at the table and have your meals together. You will find that your baby is responding to your eyes and obeying your orders.

Place a high chair next to you and place baby into it. Stay as close to your baby as possible while he feeds.

You can give your baby the same food as you are eating. Give your baby cereal for breakfast or oats. Make sure everything is sugar-free and natural. Omelets and sausages will also make a great choice. Try to have breakfast by 8 am.

At about 11 am, give your baby a light snack to munch on. This can be anything including a piece of fruit, a cup of chopped vegetables or even some nuts. These will keep the baby full and energetic until lunchtime.

Give your baby lunch by 1-1.30 pm. Lunch should be wholesome and nutritious. As a rule, fill up half the plate with vegetables and divide the rest between carbohydrates and proteins such as meat. For vegetarian babies, lentils and rice make a good choice. You can make a simple fruit salad to be eaten after lunch. Try to add 5 different colored fruits so that your baby can gain maximum benefit from eating it.

At about 4 pm, give your baby something to snack on. Small pieces of cured meat o chopped vegetables with a homemade dip will keep the baby's appetite satisfied.

Feed your baby dinner by 7 pm. Dinner has to be the lightest meal of the day. A small sandwich or some rice with lentils or beans will be sufficient.

It is wise not feed babies too close to bedtime as this can interfere with their sleep. You should leave at least a one-hour gap before bedtime.

Sleeping routine

Babies of this age will now sleep independently. You will not have to do too much toward getting your baby to sleep. You will have the chance to enjoy your free time with your spouse. But expect to have to accompany baby to his/her room for at least 6 months. Go with your child and supervise bedtime routines.

You can sing a lullaby for your baby or read a storybook. You can also recite rhymes together. Children love to enjoy the pictures in their story books.

Once your child falls asleep, wait for five minutes to ensure your baby is fully asleep. Some babies can be naughty and get up as soon as you leave. They might follow parents to their room and insist on sleeping with them. In such a case, the child should be taken back to their room and repeat the routine.

At this stage, your baby will sleep for about 10 to 12 hours per night. So if your baby goes to sleep at 8 pm, then he or she will be up at 7 am. You can wait in the room and greet your baby with a bit of encouragement.

In order to get your baby to develop the habit of sleeping alone, you must reward your baby every day. This can be in the form of praise, a hug or extra playtime.

In order to personalize the reward a bit more, you can decorate the room in whatever way pleases your baby. Incorporate your baby's favorite colors and patterns. You can also add décor that will make your baby want to sleep in his own room.

You must involve children in the process as much as possible, you must also teach them the importance of keeping the room neat by gathering their toys and putting them into their designated place.

If your baby has a sibling or siblings, then it will be a good time to make them share a room at night. You should ensure that they have separate beds, as your baby will still be too young to share a bed with another child. Try not to place your baby on the upper bunk of a bunk bed arrangement.

If your baby is unable to sleep properly with a sibling, then it would be best to separate them if possible. They can continue to sleep in your room if you have no alternative. We will look at this aspect in detail in a future chapter of this book.

Chapter 9 – Myths and Misconceptions Concerning Sleep Training

Sleep training remains one of the most important aspects of raising a baby. In this chapter, we will bust a few myths on sleep training.

Newborns are too young for sleep training

This is not true. You can start training your baby right from a young age. You do not have to wait for your baby to reach a certain age before starting with sleep training. You can start with t from the very day you bring your baby home. Remember, when babies develop their sleep habits, these continue as they get older.

Breast milk is much better than formula

This is also a myth. Although breast milk contains a lot of nutrients that are great for the baby, it might not always be the best choice. This is especially true if the mother is taking medications. Formulas contain just as much nutrition as breast milk and can nourish the baby's body quite adequately.

My baby sleeps too much. Is something wrong?

No. Nothing is wrong. All babies sleep for 17 to 20 hours during their first few weeks. This is quite normal and meant to help your baby grow stronger. Your baby is bound to wake up every 30 to 40 minutes and then go back to sleep. Your baby will not go into a state of deep sleep and will remain in the non-rapid eye movement phase. Babies will sleep less as and when they grow older.

Babies used to co-sleeping will not grow out of it

This is false. Babies can easily outgrow co-sleeping and sleep on their own in their own room. Parents can use the Ferber method (described later) to help their baby to transition. It will not take any more than a couple of months to make your baby fully independent. In fact, toddlers will prefer to sleep in their own room as they will have their privacy and also suffer less stress.

My Baby is not sleeping as much but this shouldn't bother me

This is false. It is unnatural for babies to not fall asleep during their early years. If that is occurring then there may be something wrong with the atmosphere in the bedroom. There may be too much light seeping in or it may be too noisy for your child to fall asleep. Your child may also suffer from anxiety, which can prevent him or her from falling asleep. You must address these issues as soon as possible to help your baby to sleep during the day.

My baby will sleep all day and all night

No. Most babies will sleep for a long time. This is mainly because their bodies will be growing. They will stay awake for 6 to 7 hours. You can feed them during this time and also play with them.

My baby's circadian cycle will fix itself

No. Although it might seem like your baby's circadian cycle will fix itself after a while, it is always best to help your baby out. It is quite unhealthy for your baby to reverse his or her sleep cycle. Babies have to sleep during the night and stay awake during the day as they get older. We looked at some of the measures you can adopt to achieve this in a previous chapter and it will be best to put these measures into practice straight away.

The Ferber Method is cruel

No. The Ferber method is not cruel and is only meant to help parents train their babies to sleep on their own. Your child might cry and throw a tantrum and also refuse to sleep independently. But you have to wait for this phase to pass and your baby will develop the habit of sleeping alone. The Ferber method works best with babies aged one to one and a half years old.

It is tougher to train twins

This is not true. Although twins can mean double the training, it will not always be difficult to train them. Parents can train them individually or together depending upon whatever feels convenient. It would be ideal to set and follow a schedule to train your twins so that it is easier for both you and your babies. We will look at some tips to train your twins in a future chapter of this book.

Babies cannot sleep with siblings

This is not true. Babies can indeed sleep with their siblings but need to be over the age of one year old. Babies aged one and over can share a room with a sibling or siblings or even co-sleep. In fact, they will like it better than sleeping on their own and throw less tantrums.

Babies will not sleep with their fathers

No, this is false. Babies can sleep just as well with their fathers as they can with their mothers. They will not depend on just a single parent and will sleep with both. Fathers must actively take part in raising the baby, as it will make for a great way to bond.

The above items are common misconceptions that surround sleep training.

Chapter 10 – Twins and Siblings Sleep and Co-sleeping

Parents with twins will have a tougher time, as they will have to train two children at once. Here is a guide for the parents of twins:

Twins

Twins can pose quite a challenge as they might follow different sleeping schedules and routines. Here is a simply guide to help their parents:

- Plan in advance. As soon as you get to know you are having twins, you have to begin planning.
- When it comes to feeding newborn twins, it will be best to feed them simultaneously.
- Once they reach the age of 6 months, you can change the schedule a little and feed one baby at a time when the other one is asleep.
- When it comes to sleep training, you must work with both babies at the same time. Enlist the help of your spouse or parents or someone who can rock or pat one baby to sleep.
- Make sure there is enough place for both twins to sleep comfortably and also roll around.
- Remember that your twins will have different personalities. You cannot generalize and assume that what works for one works for the other.

Siblings

- Although siblings get extremely excited at the prospect of sharing the room with a baby, it is important to wait until the child or children reach the age of one year old.

- If the sibling is much older, then he or she can help with patting or rocking the baby to sleep. But if there is only a small age difference between the two children, then you must supervise the older sibling when he or she handles the baby.
- Once baby turns 1 year old, he or she can share a bedroom with an older sibling.
- The bedroom should be spacious and the bed should be large enough to accommodate two children.
- If you are placing children in bunk beds, then the older child should be placed on the top bunk.
- You must instruct the elder sibling not to hug baby too tightly while sleeping and maintain a little distance.
- You can use a camera to keep an eye on the children.

Co-sleeping

Co-sleeping is a concept where the parents sleep with their babies in the same bed. This is often seen as a convenient way to sleep for both parents and babies. Let us take a look at the types of co-sleeping:

- Parents sleep in the same bed as babies. This type is known as bed sharing.
- Babies are made to sleep in a sidecar. This sidecar is attached to the parents' bed.
- Baby is made to sleep in a crib that is placed next to the bed

If you plan on co-sleeping with your baby then here are some tips to bear in mind:

- Always place your baby on his or her back.

- There should be enough space for the baby to roll around.
- The bed should be soft and comfortable to touch.
- There should be no gaps between the mattress and the cot or crib. It should fit correctly.
- You must use a traditional bed rather than a waterbed or recliner.
- The bed should be free from pillows, blankets, bed sheets, clothes, etc. It should be completely clear of toys.
- The bed should be against a wall and there should be no gap between the wall and the bed as baby can get trapped in the gap.

Precautions to observe

- You must avoid sleeping with your baby if you have consumed alcohol.
- If you are on medications that make you drowsy, then you must avoid co-sleeping with your baby in the same bed.
- Do not smoke and sleep next to your baby.
- Do not sleep with your baby if you have smoked.
- If you have had a long day and are extremely tired, then avoid sleeping in the same bed as your baby.
- Tie your hair back into a bun when sleeping with baby.
- Do not wear bulky clothes when sleeping next to baby.

Advantages of co-sleeping

- The biggest advantage of co-sleeping is that parents will have easy access to their babies. They will not have to get up and go to another room to pacify their baby.
- Mothers can easily feed their babies, as they will be right next to them. They will not have to get up and go to another room to feed the baby.
- In fact, it will be easier to pacify your crying baby as you can quickly feed the baby and put the baby back to sleep.

- Babies sleep better next to their parents. They will feel the warmth and sleep better. They will not wake up and cry as much during the night.
- Mothers will not have to worry about missing a feeding session and pumping the milk out. Baby can be latched easily and fed.
- Babies who co-sleep are said to be much less cranky as compared with babies who sleep in a separate room. As per studies, babies that are made to sleep in a separate room can suffer from anxiety.

Dangers of co-sleeping

- It is a big responsibility sleeping with your baby. You must be extremely careful and ensure you are taking all the right steps to keep your baby safe.
- You must not leave any room for carelessness as it can lead to injury.
- Some parents find it stressful to share a room or bed with their baby as they will feel guilty about falling asleep and taking their eyes off their baby.
- Babies too will feel some level of stress when they sleep next to their parents. The stress can also transfer between parents and children.
- Thin and underweight babies will find it difficult to co-sleep. There is also the danger of SIDS to consider.
- Co-sleeping is not ideal for premature babies.
- Babies who get used to co-sleeping find it extremely difficult to sleep in their own rooms.

Although co-sleeping comes with its share of disadvantages and advantages, you can consider starting in this manner and then shifting the baby to his or her room.

Chapter 11 – Nightmares and Sleepwalking

Nightmares and bad dreams are a part and parcel of life. Your baby is bound to experience these at some time or another. Let us take a look at why bad dreams occur and how you can deal with them:

Nightmares

Nightmares are bad dreams. These can occur at any time and it is hard to know what can trigger them.

Signs of nightmares:

There are many signs of nightmares, some of which are as follows:

- Your toddler might tell you he or she experienced a bad dream.
- Your baby or toddler will refuse to sleep and will remain uncomfortable.
- Your baby or toddler will toss and turn in the bed.
- He or she might refuse to sleep alone and may cling to you.
- Your baby might cry loudly and wake up gasping for breath.

Why nightmares occur

Nightmares can occur due to the following reasons:

- Your toddler might have read something just before sleeping that scared the child.
- Your baby or toddler might have heard a story just before sleeping that scared him or her.
- Your toddler may have watched something on TV that scared him or her.
- Your toddler may have come across a person who seems scary.
- Your toddler may have heard noises that frightened him or her.

When this occurs, talk to your child and ask what is wrong. Children might not really open up about it and it helps if you exercise patience. If your child opens up about whatever is troubling, then get rid of whatever it is that is scaring your child. It may be a book, a shadow on the window, a noise, a toy, etc. Make sure that you get rid of the problem for good. It may even be a shadow on the wall and you may be able to fix this by changing the lighting arrangement in the room.

If your toddler does not tell you what is scaring him or her, then look for the cause yourself. Try taking away one thing at a time to zero in on the culprit.

Some babies can suffer stress. This can be a result of separation anxiety, indigestion or a medical issue. If your baby is unable to get over the nightmares, then you need to consult a doctor. If the nightmares are giving the child hallucinations, this may be a sign of a fever and this is quite common with small children. In a case such as this, do not add more temperature or make the mistake of inviting the child into your bed where it is warmer as this may make the situation worse.

- Counselling your toddler can work wonders. You have to hold your toddler's hand and tell him that it is just a dream and that it will go away.
- Distract your baby as much as possible and take its mind off the stimulus. Indulge your baby in fun activities such as reading a favorite book but be careful your child does not play up just to get this extra attention. Keep your activity calm.
- Follow a relaxing routine such as giving your baby a warm bath before bedtime.
- Make sure your baby sleeps in a comfortable environment. Check the temperature in the room and ensure there is cross ventilation.
- Don't make the room too dark. Most toddlers fear the dark and assume there are hidden monsters under the bed or in the closet. You can add a light to the room that is subdued so that the child knows there is nothing there.

Sleepwalking

Sleepwalking is a phenomenon that involves sleeping walking while in a state of deep sleep. This is often seen as a problem among children that requires treatment. Also known as somnambulism, it mostly occurs in children aged 4 to 8. Most children sleepwalk within a couple of hours of falling asleep.

Most sleepwalking sessions last between 5 to 15 minutes. Although it is seen as a harmless action, it is advisable to seek help as soon as possible.

Causes of sleepwalking

- Sleepwalking can be a result of lack of sleep or tiredness.
- It can be a result of irregular sleeping habits.
- Sleepwalking can occur if your baby or toddler is ill or sick.
- Some medications containing sedatives can encourage sleepwalking.
- Sleepwalking can sometimes be as a result of hereditary causes.
- In rare cases, sleepwalking can be a result of headaches, migraines or an injury to the head.

What does sleepwalking entail?

Sleepwalking can differ from toddler to toddler. Here are some symptoms:

- Some children will sit up and repeat the same motion over and over.
- Some children will get up from bed and literally walk around the house.
- Some children mumble or talk while they are sleeping.
- The child will be in a state of deep sleep and will not respond when spoken to.
- Some children will urinate while sleepwalking.
- Some children will repeat the same actions such as opening and closing doors and windows.

Treatment

One way of preventing injury due to sleepwalking is by closing all the doors and windows and locking them tightly.

- Clearing up the floors and removing hazards that can

cause your toddler to trip up is advisable.

- Clearing out sharp objects that can harm the child may be relevant.
- Don't put the child on the top bunk of a bunk bed arrangement.
- Keep all valuable objects tucked away to avoid accidental breakage.
- Maintain ideal temperatures inside the child's bedroom.
- Don't give your child too many liquids before bed.
- Avoid giving your toddler caffeine before bed.

The sleepwalking will normally automatically stop once your child reaches 8 years of age. If you find that it does not, you can take this child to see your doctor.

Chapter 12 – The Ferber Method of Sleep Training

One of the most important aspects of sleep training is moving your baby to his or her own room. Most parents start out with co-sleeping with their babies before moving them to their own room.

One easy technique to follow is the Ferber method of sleep training. The Ferber method was devised by Richard Ferber and is one of the easiest sleep training methods to use. Alternatively known as the "cry it out" method, it is designed to help parents move their babies to their own room.

It is obvious that babies will sit up and cry out loud when they find themselves all alone in their rooms. Through natural instincts, parents will rush to their side to deal with problems and put the baby back to sleep. However, doing so will only cause babies to cry even more, often in a bid to get parents to rush in. They may see their crying as being necessary to gain the attention that they want.

According to Ferber, this is where most parents get it wrong. He advises that parents should not rush to their baby's side when the baby starts to cry but should allow the baby to "cry it out." Babies will continue crying for some time but do fall asleep once they realize their parents are not going to come in and pacify them. Although it sounds a little savage, it is a great way to get children to fall asleep by themselves.

The Ferber method is quite strict and required you to follow a set schedule. You must set a proper feeding and sleeping schedule for your baby and follow it religiously in order for the method to work.

- First, rock or pat your baby and lay the baby into the crib. Your baby should be sleepy but not asleep. Babies should be laid down on their backs. Leave the room when baby is still awake and looking at you. The baby will start to whimper. Then the baby will try to get your attention by crying.

- When this happens, you have to remain patient and not rush into the room. You have to wait for 5 to 10 minutes before entering the room again and pacifying your baby. Once the child is silent again, you must place the baby into the crib as before and leave the room.
- Continue doing this for 30 minutes by which time your baby should fall asleep.
- You must continue with this technique for about a month and a half.
- Many parents give up on the method and feel like it is cruel to let their babies cry so much. However, it will get better with time and your baby will stop crying.
- You can install cameras in the room to keep an eye on your baby from a distance. That way, you will know whether your baby is up to mischief or has any difficulty that needs to be addressed.
- The crib should be cleared of all items including toys, bottles, pillows, blankets, etc. These can pose a threat to your baby's health.
- Once your baby is accustomed to it, you can read baby a story and give him/her a kiss goodnight.

Here is a simply timetable to follow to train your baby using the Ferber Method:

1. Day 1 – 3 minutes 1st interval – 5 minutes 2nd interval – 10 minutes 3rd interval, 10 minutes – remaining intervals.
2. Day 2 – 5 minutes 1st interval – 10 minutes 2nd interval – 12 minutes 3rd interval – 12 minutes remaining intervals.
3. Day 3 – 10 minutes 1st interval – 12 minutes 2nd interval – 15 minutes 3rd interval – 15 minutes remaining intervals.
4. Day 4 – 12 minutes 1st interval – 15 minutes 2nd interval – 17 minutes 3rd interval – 17 minutes remaining intervals.
5. Day 5 – 15 minutes 1st interval – 17 minutes 2nd interval – 20 minutes 3rd interval – 20 minutes remaining intervals.
6. Day 6 – 17 minutes 1st interval – 20 minutes 2nd interval – 25 minutes 3rd interval – 25 minutes remaining intervals.
7. Day 7 – 20 minutes 1st interval – 25 minutes 2nd interval – 30 minutes 3rd interval – 30 minutes remaining intervals.

Pros of the Ferber Method

- The Ferber Method is one of the most preferred sleep training methods in the world. It is used to train babies to fall asleep on their own. It is simple and very effective.

- The Ferber Method is designed to be flexible. You can choose to follow whatever timings suit your baby's needs. Once babies get accustomed to it, they will fall asleep on their own with little difficulty.

- The Ferber Method is quite effective and works on your baby in express time. This means that you do not have to worry about losing sleep over your baby's tantrums.

- According to research, babies trained using the Ferber Method are less likely to be cranky. They will sleep well and develop a healthy mind and body.

- The Ferber Method will help parents sleep better as well.

Cons of the Ferber Method

- The majority of parents who fail with this method give up on the Ferber Method very soon after they start it. They will not give it a fair chance and think of it as a savage way of training their baby to fall asleep.

- Some babies will develop separation anxiety and fear going to bed. It might take a very long time for them to adjust to it and they can give their parents sleepless nights.

These form the pros and cons of the Ferber Method. However, most people agree that this method is effective and you can use it to train your baby to sleep on his or her own. When tending your baby during the intervals between crying, try to keep sound at a minimum and help the baby to associate the whole process with night time sleeping. Getting angry and frustrated will not help parents or the child.

Chapter 13 – Dealing with Travel

Traveling is a fun activity that children enjoy. But it proves to be a hassle for parents, as they have to take care of the many aspects involved in travel. In this chapter, we look at some tips to follow to make traveling with your baby a breeze.

- Always plan out your trips in advance. That way, you will have enough time to sketch out a sleeping schedule for your baby. Remember that your baby's sleep cycle should not be disturbed during travel and should remain the same as when the child is at home.

- Make a list of everything that your baby will need on the trip and pack it well in advance. Doing this last minute can make you forget something important.

- Write down the times when your baby takes a nap during the daytime and nighttime. You must follow the same routine when you are traveling.

- You have to buy a crib to place your baby in during the car ride. The crib has to be safe and comfortable for your baby. Take the baby along when buying one so that you can test it out for size and comfort.

- Not all babies will find traveling convenient and some will cry quite a bit. You must prepare yourself for this and use a pacifier to help them to stop crying.

- One good way to help babies to sleep while in motion is

by holding them as close to your body as possible and gently rock them. You can partially cover their eyes with a blanket if there is too much light, but do make sure that it does not cover their nose or mouth.

- It will be a good idea to open the windows partially to allow fresh air into the car. Your baby should be able to inhale fresh air, but do keep babies away from drafts and cold air.

- If you have been driving for a long time, then step out for a short while to take some fresh air. Your baby or toddler will also need the break. For those traveling by plane, walk with your baby up and down the aisle.

- Playing soft, soothing music can help your baby to sleep better. Let the music play whenever the baby needs to sleep and ask those in the car to keep noise to a minimum during this time.

- Take your baby on smaller trips to accustom the child to traveling in the car. Traveling far without practice might prove to be extremely tedious for your baby or toddler. Take your child out every alternate day for a week to ensure that travel is not stressful.

- Take turns to drive if you are driving long distance. Plan it out in such a way that you and your partner both have equal time behind the wheel or with the baby.

- Make sure you carry your baby's favorite toys and blankets. The baby will take comfort from the familiarity of these objects. Play with the child the same way as you do at home and follow the same schedule that you have already established.

Following these tips can help you to have a smooth journey with your baby.

Chapter 14 – Babies with Colic and Other Issues Faced by Parents

It is obvious that not all children will be the same. Some will require extra care and attention, as their needs will be different from others. In this chapter, we look at what colic is and what parents can do about it. We will also shed light on some of the issues that parents can face while raising their babies.

What is Colic?

Collis is a condition where your baby will cry for no apparent reason. It is a fact that all babies will cry as it is their number one resort to seek attention or satisfy a need. But those babies that cry without any reason are said to suffer from colic. Although it might seem strange that some babies cry more than others, it only goes to show that not all babies are the same.

Colic is not an illness or disease that needs a cure. Rather, it is a condition that requires treatment. Here are some criteria that qualify crying as colic:

- The crying is abrupt and your baby cries for no apparent reason.
- The crying lasts for 3 to 4 hours at a stretch.
- The crying may last daily over a period of 3 to 4 weeks.
- The baby cries at the same time each day.
- Your baby clenches fists and starts flailing legs while crying.
- Your baby spits out while crying.
- Your baby starts to cry while eating or sleeping.

If you notice any of these signs, then chances are high your baby is suffering from colic. Here are some of the causes of colic:

- Colic can be set off due to hyperactive senses. Some babies might not be able to control the response to a certain stimuli and end of feeling agitated and start crying.
- Babies with a weak digestive system can end up developing colic. They will not be able to control the changes in their bodies.
- Some babies can suffer from GERD, which causes acid reflux. This can make them restless and cranky.
- Some babies can have food allergies. These can be manifested by colic.
- Babies who are exposed to smoking or any tobacco products can develop colic.
- Babies exposed to strong smells can also develop colic.

Solutions for colic

- If your baby has colic, then you must calm the baby. Pick baby up and rock or pat the baby. Your baby will feel more relaxed when he or she is in your arms.
- Check to see what is exciting your baby so much. If you find out what appears to trigger the attacks, you can then control them.
- Babies who are crying owing to indigestion should be taken to the doctor. The doctor will be able to decide whether to prescribe any medications to help to relieve gas and indigestion.
- Use white noise to help calm your baby down. White noise or even calming music can work wonders on your

baby and you can find some of this kind of music on YouTube if you are unsure about what it is.

- Give your baby his or her favorite pacifier to control the crying.
- If nothing seems to work, then allow the colic to subside on its own. As per studies, colic does not last for that long and will subside as your baby reaches a certain age. However, do rule out any medical reasons your baby may be suffering by talking with your doctor if the baby's discomfort levels seem abnormal.

Other Issues

Sleeplessness

One of the biggest challenges faced by new parents is not getting enough sleep. It is obvious that babies will wake up at odd and anti-social hours and eat away into parents' sleep. This can lead to all types of issues including anxiety and, in some cases, depression. It is best for parents to find some sort of escape so that they do not feel overwhelmed by the experience. Sleeplessness can also affect physical health and so it would be ideal for parents to take turns to tend to the baby and get as much sleep as possible.

Nighttime feeding

Babies need food both in the morning and at night. New mothers find it especially difficult to feed babies at night time. In such a case, it would be ideal to pump milk out in advance and use this to feed the baby. In fact, the father can feed the baby using a bottle. It is also a good idea to feed your baby formula if you are unable to get up as often. You can mix formula and keep it ready so that your partner can feed the baby.

Feeding Schedule

Not all babies will feed the same way thereby making it tough for parents to set a schedule. Some babies might feed every 2 hours while others might feed every hour. You must set a schedule based on how often your baby likes to be fed. If you already have experience of feeding a baby, then you can try the same schedule with the newborn.

Teething trouble

Toddlers undergoing teething will put an end of their parents' sleep. Teething can be quite painful and make it impossible for parents to sleep owing to all the crying. During this phase, parents have to take in turns to pacify the toddler. Keep teething toys handy so that they can be given to the baby as soon as he or she starts to cry. Teething can last a long time thereby making it quite difficult for parents to carry out routine activities. Parents will have to remain patient through it in order to avoid unnecessary stress.

Dirty work

One of the most important aspects to prepare for is the dirty work. This includes changing the diapers and cleaning up the vomit. Changing diapers is generally seen as a Herculean task, but does not have to be that way. You can watch online videos on how to fasten a diaper or use pant style diapers. Both mother and father should know how to do it, so that they can share the workload. If you tap your baby's back after eating, then you can expect your child to throw up. You have to prepare for this and have some tissues or a cloth handy so that it can be cleaned up straight away.

Toddler Tantrums

It is easier to control babies, as they will not be able to do too many things on their own. However, raising a toddler is a whole new ball game as they will be much more independent and inquisitive. You will have to prepare yourself to put up with a lot of tantrums and remain on your toes. Toddlers are bound to be mischievous and indulge in activities that can land them in trouble. You must prepare yourself for all types of situations and remain proactive. This will be especially tedious if you have twins or a baby has a young sibling. You and your spouse will have to take turns to keep an eye on the baby or enlist the help of a sitter or family member to take care of the baby.

Working parents

Some working parents feel guilty about leaving their baby behind. They will not be able to work properly owing to guilt. In such a case, it would be better for parents to wait until their baby is grown sufficiently. Working parents who take care of their babies and stay up at night will also find it difficult to go to work in the morning and tend to get irritable. It is therefore best to wait until baby reaches a more manageable age before rejoining the workforce.

Conclusion

I thank you once again for choosing this look and hope you had a good time reading it. The main aim of the book was to educate you on the basics of sleep training of your baby.

Sleep is one of the most important aspects of life. Your baby will develop a healthy body and lead a happy life if he or she gets enough sleep during the growing up years. Although it will require a little compromise on your part, it will be well worth it. You will have an enjoyable time raising your little ones and developing a lasting bond with them.

I thank you once again and wish you all the best!

Finally, if you enjoyed this book, then I would like to ask you a favor. Would you be kind enough to leave a review of this book on Amazon? It would be greatly appreciated.

Thank you and good luck!

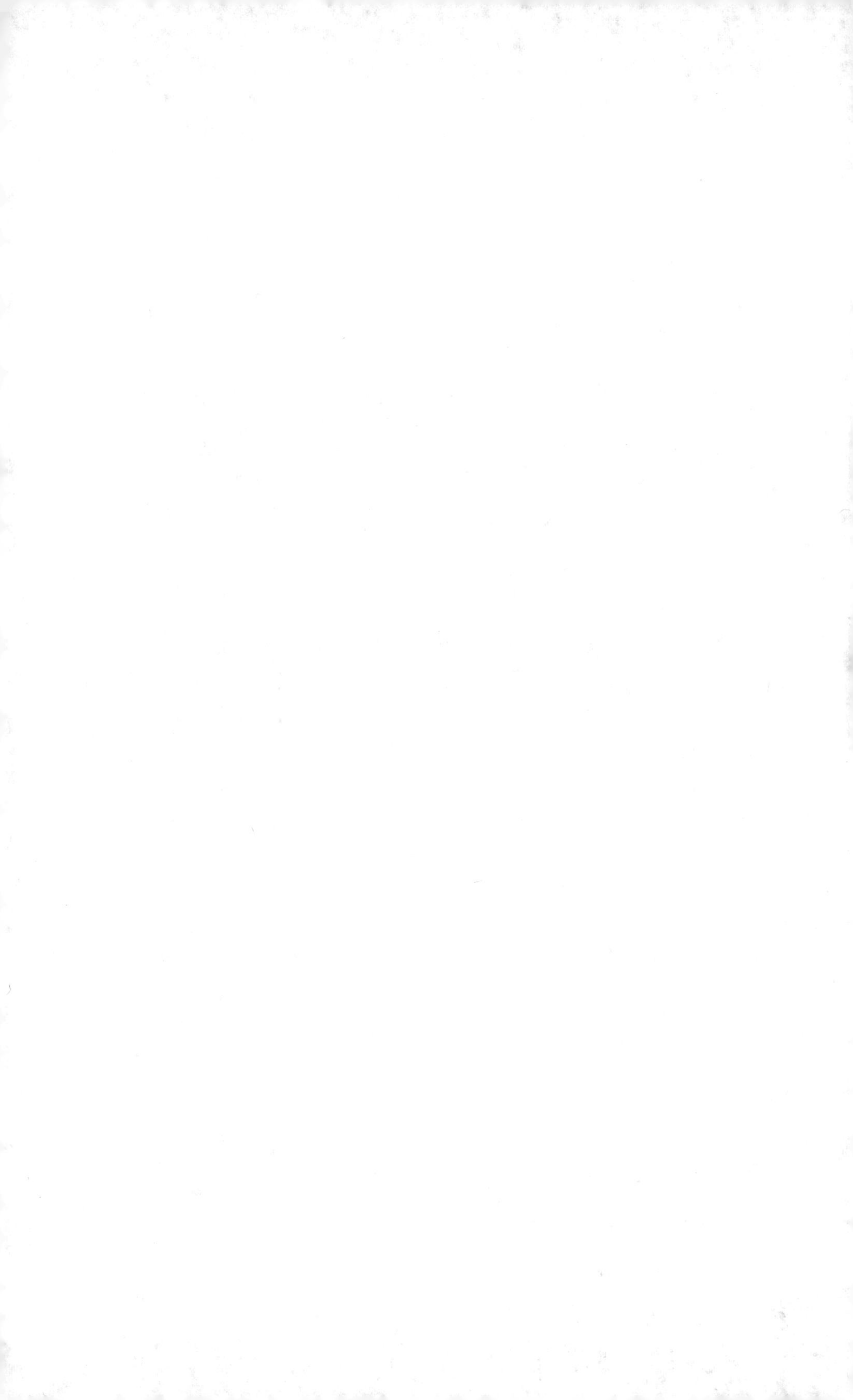